VOLUME 73

THE CHEMISTRY OF CANCER

TAUTOMERISM AND METHYLATION

FINAL EDITION AUGUST 2022

Carlos L Partidas

DEDICATION

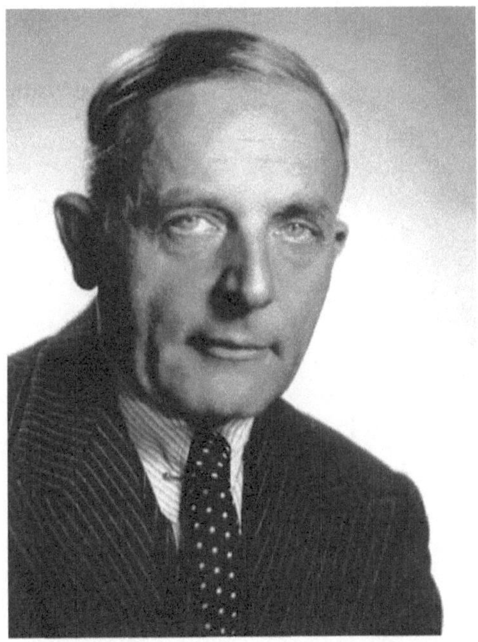

German physiologist and biochemist Otto Heinrich Warburg, who discovered that cancer cells live in an acidic environment without oxygen

TABLE OF CONTENTS

ACKNOWLEDGEMENT

LIVING BEINGS, WHO LIVE IN THIS PHYSICAL STATION OF THE
ENERGY LEVELS, TO BE TEMPORARILY ON EARTH

Chapter 1

ACID-BASE BALANCE

To produce caloric energy, the mitochondria of healthy cells can achieve this with the sugar glucose and oxygen. Glucose comes from carbohydrates via food, and oxygen from respiration via haemoglobin transport. After the generation of energy, carbon dioxide will be generated in the mitochondria as a waste product. However, if no oxygen arrives via respiration because haemoglobin is blocked due to acidosis caused by uric acid, the mitochondria will resort to the process of glucose fermentation, also known as glycolysis. When energy production in the form of heat goes via glycolysis, lactate will be generated in the mitochondria instead of carbon dioxide.

In healthy cells, the mitochondria use these two pathways to produce heat energy, as the process will depend on how the cellular respiration of each living thing is adapted: for example, when we were a germ, there was no oxygen in the mitochondria in the tails of the sperm. At that time, the sugar for energy production was fructose. By breaking down fructose, not lactate but glucose and galactose are generated. Thus, fructose is the sugar that is present in the gonads in haploid form in all male mammals.

When the sperm is introduced into the other haploid, i.e. the egg, replication will continue until ageing; passing through the stages of an embryo and a baby in the womb until birth occurs. The cells of the embryo need glucose and oxygen to replicate; therefore, these two substances are present in the mother's blood where the embryo grows, and from the mother's blood, the embryo will take the necessary nutrients for cell growth or replication. For the respiration of its cells in the womb, the baby will use the glucose and oxygen provided by the mother.

Thus, the supply of nutrients to the embryo will depend on the mother's respiration and the kind of food she eats. If no oxygen reaches the mitochondria of the foetus' cells, the mitochondria will resort to the process of fermentation. However, this will no longer be by fermentation of fructose, but by glycolysis of glucose. Thus, lactate will be generated by this route of respiration.

Through sleep, there will be more oxygen; and lactate will be converted back to pyruvate and pyruvate will be converted back to glucose. So, the life of the embryo, and as the embryo grows into a baby in the womb, the respiration of its cells will be by the normal oxygen-glucose pathway, which depends on the mother's breathing and food.

After birth, nourishment has to come from the mother's milk. In the mother's milk, the sugar is lactose. From lactose the baby can get the sugars glucose and galactose. From glucose, the baby can get the caloric energy in the mitochondria of its cells, while from the sugar galactose, the baby can get the basic nutrients for the continued formation of the nervous system.

Initially, the newborn does not produce enough saliva in the mouth, so in order to obtain from the mother's milk these compounds necessary for energy and the strengthening of the nervous system from galactose, the baby has the enzyme lactase in its small intestine. The enzyme lactase begins to disappear when the baby produces saliva in the mouth, as the enzyme amylase allows the baby to obtain glucose from the breakdown of carbohydrates in food. While oxygen will continue to be obtained through respiration, where the process will depend on the degree of acidity of the blood.

In the alveoli, the degree of acidity is lower, so that carbonic acid is broken down into water vapour and carbon dioxide. The carbonic acid was transported from the periphery of the cells by haemoglobin. Haemoglobin has four heme groups; and each heme group is bonded to an oxygen atom. Thus, when the heme group is left empty after exhalation, haemoglobin binds with 4 oxygen molecules in the alveoli and carries them to the cell periphery.

What causes haemoglobin to carry oxygen into the cells and transport carbonic acid to the lungs is a change in the degree of acidity. In the inner part of the cells, the acidity value is neutral, i.e. the pH is 7.00; whereas, in the lungs the acidity value is 7.40. This acidity range has to be narrow, so that it is the same haemoglobin molecule that transports oxygen from the lungs to the periphery of the cell and takes carbonic acid from the periphery of the cell to the lungs.

In the periphery of the cells, the acidity is higher; therefore, haemoglobin exchanges with myoglobin the oxygen brought from the lungs for the carbonic acid produced by the mitochondria inside the cells. Myoglobin has only one heme group, which is why myoglobin is smaller than haemoglobin. Myoglobin is more abundant in the blood relative to the amount of haemoglobin. Because it is smaller than haemoglobin, myoglobin can enter the cells to carry oxygen to the mitochondria. Myoglobin is red in colour, and because it is more abundant, myoglobin is the reserve of oxygen for the cells. Myoglobin is the substance that gives blood its red colour.

In the cell periphery, haemoglobin binds carbonic acid preferentially with oxygen, because in the cell periphery, the acid value is higher than in the lungs.

The reductive system inside cells with normal acidity prevents the acidity level from increasing inside the cell.

If the blood becomes acidic, the haemoglobin cannot be released from the carbonic acid; therefore, there is no oxygen transport to the mitochondria of the cells. If there is no oxygen in the mitochondria, the mitochondria will produce energy by the second route, i.e. by fermentation of glucose. However, if the acidity inside the cells is high, lactate will be produced instead of pyruvate. If the acidity remains high inside the cell, lactate will be converted to lactic acid.

The enzyme carbonic anhydrase is responsible for converting carbon dioxide into carbonic acid. In this reaction, a high acidity is produced in the cytoplasm, as a proton is released into the reductive system inside the cell. The reductive system within the cell will ensure that the degree of acidity does not increase, as without the reductive system, lactate would be converted to lactic acid. Lactic acid inside the cell would damage the cellular reductive system. Among them, the enzyme carbonic anhydrase will cease to function, so that myoglobin will not be able to bring oxygen into the cells, but neither will myoglobin be able to take the waste out of the cell as carbonic acid if the reductive system inside the cells is damaged.

If the degree of acidity is higher inside the cell, the nucleus of the cell will be affected, as the hydrogen bonds between the bases forming the DNA will be modified. As a result, chromosomes will insert base pairs incorrectly, due to two associated effects, tautomerism and methylation.

There must be a balance inside and outside the cell. For example, outside the cell, a reducing enzyme system is needed for NAD to reduce haemoglobin iron III to iron II, but it is NAD itself that oxidises haemoglobin iron II to iron III. So, that myoglobin can take out carbonic acid from the cells as iron III. In order for haemoglobin to carry oxygen to the periphery of the cell, the iron in haemoglobin has to be in the form of iron II. In turn, in order for myoglobin to carry oxygen to the inner part of the cells, the oxidation state of the iron in myoglobin has to be as iron II.

Then, on the outside of the cell, the acidity is high, so the process is reversed: the myoglobin releases the carbonic acid and captures the oxygen released by the haemoglobin, when the haemoglobin binds with the carbonic acid. The bloodstream pulls the haemoglobin back into the lungs to carry the carbonic acid out of the body.

This is the process for normal respiration that takes place inside and outside the cells. But this system of exchanging carbon dioxide for oxygen does not correspond to a chemical reaction, but to a process of exchanging oxygen for carbonic acid. This is why Dr. Max Ferdinand Perutz called it the cooperative effect.

It is to Dr. Perutz that we owe the description of the respiratory process in cells. Although Dr. Perutz based the description of cellular respiration on the measurement of the oxygen partial pressure value of 100 mm of mercury in the lungs and 40 mm of mercury in the muscle, these were the variables that Dr. Ferdinand Perutz could measure. But, we deduce, that the change of these values is rather due to a change of acidity than to a change of oxygen partial pressure.

The higher acidity value outside the cell is called the Bohr effect. The description of the process is due to the Danish physicist Niels Henrik David Bohr.

The subsequent experimental analysis of Dr. Ferdinand Perutz is based on the observation of the German scientist Otto Heinrich Warburg that cancer cells reproduce in an acidic medium and an oxygen-free environment.

Acidity outside the normal range is caused by an increased concentration of uric acid in the blood. The increased uric acid concentration in the blood is due to the consumption of cells of animal origin. All organisms, at least mammals, are consubstantial, so that our cells are chemically the same as those of other animals. The only thing that makes us look physically different is the order in which these bases are inserted in the DNA, i.e. the genetic code.

After birth, this narrow range of acidity for the process of respiration inside and outside the cells can be modified by food, mainly due to a lack of knowledge of the respiratory process of exchanging oxygen for carbonic acid. Depending on the type of food ingested, we can produce a change in the coupling of the bases in DNA.

The change in the coupling of the bases in DNA is what is known as a mutation, which will give rise to cancer. It is a mutation because the modification of DNA occurs through the effect of tautomerism and methylation of electronic matter.

The correct or incorrect coupling of these bases in DNA, adenine-thymine, thymine-cytokine and guanine ketone-cytokine, is going to depend on the chemistry inside the nucleus and in the chromosomes of the cells. So, the chemistry inside and outside our cells will ultimately depend on us, because we are the ones who decide how we feed ourselves. And the way we feed ourselves as adults is a voluntary act.

We are going to look mathematically at the range or value of sodium urate and uric acid concentrations to show why and how sodium urate is converted into uric acid, which is a consequence of the mutations that occur in the cells. Or we can use this relationship to check the proportions of uric acid and sodium urate in the normal blood of a healthy person and in a person with cancer by means of the following formula:

$$[\text{sodium urate}] = 10^{(pH\text{-}pka)} [\text{uric acid}]$$

The pka of uric acid is 5.8; therefore, substituting the values for the pH value of a person whose blood has a normal acidity value or pH equal to 7.40 we have that:

$$[\text{sodium urate}] = 10^{7.4\text{-}5.8} [\text{uric acid}].$$

$$[\text{sodium urate}] = 10^{1.6} [\text{uric acid}]$$

$$[\text{sodium urate}] = 40 [\text{uric acid}]$$

In other words, for the blood of a person whose blood acidity value is normal, the sodium urate concentration should be approximately 40 times higher than the uric acid concentration.

Whereas, for the blood of a person involved with a terminal case of cancer, the pH of the blood is 5.5; thus, this relationship is:

$$[\text{sodium urate}] = 10^{5.5-5.8}\,[\text{uric acid}]$$

$$[\text{sodium urate}] = 10^{-0.3}\,[\text{uric acid}]$$

$$[\text{sodium urate}] = 0.5\,[\text{uric acid}]$$

Which indicates that, if the blood is too acidic for a person with a terminal case of cancer, the concentration of uric acid in this case doubles, i.e. the concentration of uric acid is twice as high as the concentration of sodium urate:

$$[\text{uric acid}] = 2\,[\text{sodium urate}]$$

In other words, in the blood of a person with end-stage cancer, there will no longer be the antioxidant sodium urate, or perhaps any other antioxidant available, to reduce iron in haemoglobin from ferric ion III to ferrous ion II; therefore, there will be no oxygen transport, as haemoglobin is neutralised by carbonic acid.

Most likely, this high acidity will also affect the antioxidant NAD^+ and NADH. Because, if the acidity value in a person with terminal cancer is 4.5, the ratio [sodium urate]/[uric acid] will be higher. And in this cancer case, the uric acid concentration would be more than twice as high as the sodium urate concentration.

So, if the acidity is high, all the healthy cells will be starved of oxygen, because the haemoglobin is blocked by the uric acid. So, the whole set of cells of the person with cancer would be paralysed by lack of oxygenation.

There will be an acme or paroxysm in the person with a more acidic blood environment, where the rest of the healthy cells fold; because, the healthy cells will not be able to take up oxygen to survive. Whereas the cancer cells changed the form of existence of the healthy person, forced by the magnetic mass of the spirit that only temporarily resides in a body made of electronic matter, which was not configured to ingest the flesh of another animal as food. The normal process can be modified without knowledge, for the matter of the cells forming the electronic body is only electronic energy condensed into the form of electronic matter. In other words, the electronic matter of the body is changeable. Therefore, this is the only kind of electronic matter that can adapt to the changes induced in the living being.

The conditions have been achieved, so that both kinds of cancer cells and mutant cells can no longer coexist in the same body. And these conditions of higher acidity are favourable only for the survival of the mutant cells, because these mutated cells can survive without oxygen, as the German physiologist Otto Heinrich Warburg analysed.

If there is no oxygen, this situation is not favourable for those cells that are still healthy. This will happen, until the anomaly of high acidity, which is caused by the imbalance, or as a consequence of the low pH value, i.e. the high acidity of the body, is reversed in time. As long as we do not find a way to lower the acidosis, we have no other way to reverse the cancer condition.

It is a successful strategy to change the way some people with cancer eat, because they have changed their lifestyle in time from being carnivores to being vegetarians, and they have been relieved of the disease, even in those people with end-stage cancer. Because perhaps, with this change of dietary strategy, if the change is timely, they have succeeded in restoring the blood that had become acidic to its normal acid value. Perhaps because they have understood in time that what causes the damage is the consumption of meat, which contains the cells that cause acidity and then tautomerism. Meanwhile, the proteins that meat also contains induce methylation of the cytokine bases and uracil, when the uracil base has changed from ketonic to enolic.

The only way to give the cells that remain healthy a new chance is for the cells themselves to regain control of their chemical balance, or the ideal condition of functioning, by their own autonomy, or perhaps by trying not to force all the cells to be affected in a process of metastasis.

We conclude that the origin of cancer is due to an acid-alkali imbalance in the blood, which can be reversed chemically, but not with a vaccine. Because the case of cancer is not an immunological but a chemical problem. And the pathological differences in this anomaly are due to the kind of epithelial tissue involved, because 80% of cancer cases originate in epithelial tissue, mainly in the apical cells. Apical cells have no blood supply of their own, and the nutrition of these apical cells depends on the cells that form the underlying epithelial tissue.

Examples of these are the apical cells of the milk ducts in the breast, the apical cells in the seminal vesicles connected to the prostate, the apical cells of the skin that are exposed to the external environment, and the glial cells of the brain, which assist neurons with nutrients. Neurons are dedicated to electronic conduction; therefore, neurons have no blood supply pathways.

The impairment of glial cells in the brain due to lack of oxygenation can lead to Alzheimer's disease or Parkinson's disease. The other factor contributing to the lack of oxygenation of glial cells in the brain is blood viscosity. When the blood becomes more viscous, the fluidity decreases; and what can increase the viscosity of the blood is the consumption of dairy products.

There will additionally be a problem known as anorexic cancer, which manifests itself in those with end-stage cancer. In this advanced stage of cancer, there will be an increased lack of appetite; and the listlessness due to lack of oxygenation will cause the affected person to run out of energy. So, the cancer sufferer will fall into a more frequent state of sleep, and then this lack of oxygen will become the main cause of the disconnection of the mass of the spirit from the electronic matter of the body. Perhaps the disconnection was not due to the cancer itself, but the lack of interest in food and the hopelessness of the health condition will create this indisposition, apathy or listlessness, which will worsen the countenance of the person affected by cancer.

The second most important antioxidant in the blood after sodium urate is vitamin C; and because it is water-soluble, we lose vitamin C through urine and perspiration. Therefore, we will need to obtain vitamin C from fruit consumption. Whereas we do not need to consume the cells of another animal to obtain sodium urate from them, as we get this antioxidant in abundance from our own cells that are no longer functioning. It is from the purine adenine and guanine bases of our DNA and the various extinct RNAs that we will obtain our antioxidant sodium urate.

By a seemingly insignificant change in the acidity value between the renal fluid and the blood a proper balance of both sodium urate and uric acid is maintained, which has to move within a range of concentration, which is determined by a constant called the dissociation or equilibrium constant; i.e.:

$$K_{eq}= [\text{sodium urate}] \times [\text{protons}]/ [\text{uric acid}].$$

The concentration of sodium urate is:

$$[\text{sodium urate}]= K_{eq} [\text{uric acid}] / [\text{protons}]$$

The quantity between the brackets is read as concentration.

It means, that the dissociation constant of uric acid K_{eq} in the blood has to be very large, or that the uric acid must be almost completely dissociated in the form of sodium urate, so that the concentration of protons remains constant. That is, in order for the concentration of these substances to remain within a narrow range of pH values, because this range should be neither above 7.45 nor below 7.35, i.e. in reality this pH value has to oscillate around 7.40. If this acidity value falls below 7.35, the problems of acidosis arise. Whereas, if the pH value is above 7.45, another problem called alkalosis will arise.

But both problems, acidosis or alkalosis, are only determined by the value of this equilibrium constant, which is related to the concentration of protons in the blood. Because if the value of the proton concentration moves towards higher values, the equilibrium value will also change in order to keep the ratio within a new value, i.e. the range of sodium urate and uric acid concentrations. In this case, in order to keep the value of the ratio constant, the uric acid concentration will become larger.

The cancer problem, of course, can be reversed chemically, as soon as we can lower the concentration of protons and uric acid in the blood. If we somehow managed to keep this balance within the value at which the cells function normally, cancer would not occur, of course, because there is no organic reason for this to happen.

Chapter 2

TAUTOMERISM

The tautomerism effect refers to a change of electronic configuration that happens to a ketone to become an alcohol. As can be seen in Figure 6, in the case of the ketone guanine base, which is transformed into an alcoholic guanine. If tautomerism occurs to a ketone, it will cause the couplings between the bases to change, thus changing the electronic structure of DNA. In DNA, the ketone bases most prone to tautomerism are the guanine and uracil bases.

The guanine base can change from its normal ketonic form to its tautomer or alcoholic form. Whereas, the uracil base, after losing its beta hydrogen, can switch from its ketonic form to its alcoholic configuration. When it loses its beta hydrogen, the uracil base will lose the alpha hydrogen that is on nitrogen number 3; and when it loses this alpha hydrogen, an enolic uracil base will undergo a methylation process. To locate which is the uracil nitrogen 3, look at Figure 5.

In this case of tautomerism, the enolic guanine base can readjust the shape of its coupling under the effect of acidosis, which is an electronic process. Whereas, in the methylation process, both the uracil base from its enolic form and the cytosine base will be converted to the thymine base, and thus the cytokine and uracil bases disappear from the cell nucleus.

To form DNA, the chromosomes will continue to pair the adenine base with the thymine base; but, once the cytosine and uracil bases disappear from the cell nucleus, the chromosomes will have to pair the enolic guanine base with the thymine base. This DNA will be wrong in its electronic configuration; or let's say, this DNA does not correspond to the original DNA that configured the cells of a human being, before its bases underwent the process of tautomerism and methylation, as a consequence of the increase of the degree of acidity in the nucleus of the cells.

Tautomerism comes from the consumption of cells of animal origin, as the adenine and guanine purine bases in the DNA of the ingested cells will be converted to sodium urate. But, if there is acidosis in the blood, the sodium urate will be transformed into enolic uric acid. At normal acidity, the form of uric acid is ketonic. Enolic uric acid is a stronger acid than ketonic uric acid. For example, ketonic uric acid does not attack calcium in the bones; but, enolic uric acid will strip calcium from the cartilage that forms part of the joints, leading to deformed arthritis and osteoporosis.

As mentioned, in order to maintain a balance between the concentration of sodium urate and uric acid in the blood, excess sodium urate, or urate from consumed cells, will have to be converted to enolic uric acid, according to the following balance equation:

$$[uric\ acid] \leftrightarrow [sodium\ urate] + [protons]$$

This equation shows that, when there is a high concentration of sodium urate in the blood, in order to maintain chemical equilibrium between the amounts of sodium urate and H^+ protons, the concentration of uric acid has to increase. Whereas, the high concentration of H^+ protons on the right will reach a point at which it can no longer be regulated by the buffering system of the blood. That is, by the sodium carbonate $\leftrightarrow$ carbonic acid buffer system, whose buffering capacity controls the blood acidity value so that it does not go outside its normal range, which is between a pH value of 7.35 and 7.45. For the acidity to remain within its normal functional range or value, the pH must be 7.40. So, if there is an increase in the acidity value, the balance will move towards a higher range of H^+ proton concentration, i.e. of enolic uric acid.

This regulatory system is known as a buffer, and in this case, the sodium carbonate came from the sodium chloride consumed with the meal, when the sodium chloride salt was converted into stomach acid by the enzyme secretin. The function of stomach acid is to activate the enzyme pepsin so that it degrades the proteins that were ingested with the meal. Proteins must be broken down in the stomach during digestion, so that the amino acids that make up the protein reach the cells in free form. In cells, the amino acids bind to transfer RNA, so that ribosomes insert them one by one, according to the triplet that brings the messenger RNA from the nucleus, for the ribosomes to build the different proteins.

The enzyme pepsin is inactivated in the form of pepsinogen so that pepsin does not attack the proteins in the stomach. If pepsin is not inactivated, gastric ulceration can occur in the duodenum, as the duodenum is highly acidic, because it is in the duodenum that the chyme produced during digestion is neutralised. The chyme is neutralised by the bile fluid.

The degree of acidity in the small intestine from the pyloric valve in the duodenum must be alkaline so that carbon dioxide gas bubbles do not form with the hydrochloric acid in the stomach. This can lead to other consequences, such as refluxes that can cause belching from the carbon dioxide gas that forms, and the dragging of bile fluids into the oesophagus or gastritis.

The other purpose of neutralising chyme by bile salts in the duodenum is for the enzymes trypsin and chymotrypsin to continue the degradation of the peptides or protein remnants that could not be degraded during stomach digestion; these are degraded to a lower degree of acidity. Generally, these peptides that were not degraded in the stomach consist of aromatic amino acids, which are more difficult to degrade at high acidity.

By the consumption of animal cells, the acidity value of the blood will move out of its functional range, and thus the blood pH decreases, i.e. the acidity of the blood increases.

But no matter what kind of animal flesh is consumed; be it cow, sheep, chicken or fish; they are all living beings made up of cells; and, apart from what we have said, that we are all formed by magnetic matter in the form of spirits; that is, the energy that gives vitality to the changing electronic matter of the body of any living being. Both energies are produced by the movement of the Universe; thus, all living beings are siblings both genetically and energetically.

When uric acid accumulates in the blood, it begins to release calcium from the bones, and calcium urate will form; but, once the calcium urate passes through the acidic environment of the kidneys into the urinary bladder, the calcium urate will crystallise and gallstones and kidney stones will form.

Protein consumed with the piece of meat brings with it an excess of the amino acid methionine, which, losing its methyl group, is converted to homocysteine and will lead to methylation of the enolic uracil and cytokine. If there is acidosis, the uracil from its ketone form will change to its enolic form; and from the enolic form, the uracil will undergo, like the cytosine base, a methylation process. The result of this methylation process is that both the cytosine and uracil bases will become the thymine base.

Tautomerism causes the shapes of the base couplings in DNA and RNA to be altered. This fact is verifiable, since it is in the enolic form that uric acid crystals are formed in the joints of arthritic people. To be more precise, this uric acid in the joints of arthritics is the one found in the kidneys, and is actually in the form of 3-methyluric acid, i.e. uric acid in arthritics is in the enolic form.

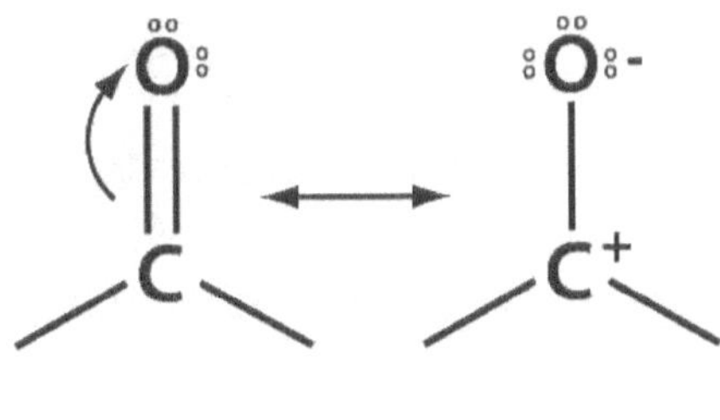

FIGURE 1

HIGH ACIDITY CONVERTS THE CARBONYL GROUP OF A KETONE =C=O ON THE LEFT TO AN ALCOHOL ≡C-OH ON THE RIGHT

The process of tautomerism is chemical; therefore, we have no other way to explain it. So, try to invest some effort to understand it in this chapter. As we have said, the phenomenon of tautomerism occurs when a ketone becomes an alcohol, because in an acidic environment, alcohols are more stable than ketones.

Although the double bond of the ketone (=C=O) on the left of Figure 1 is stable, (~178 kcal/mol) it is only slightly stronger than the single bond ($\equiv$C-OH) of the alcohol on the right (~2 x 85.5 kcal/mol). For this to happen, certain conditions are required: for example, there must be a hydrogen H next to the carbonyl group (=C=O) so that it can detach and compensate for the positive charge generated on the carbon atom ($\equiv$C$^+$). It is this hydrogen that is called alpha hydrogen, because it is the one that is closest to the carbonyl group. This is the alpha hydrogen that can leave, so that the ketone can be converted into an alcohol, that is, so that the ketone can undergo a tautomerism process. The next hydrogen that is prone to leave would be beta hydrogen, which is the hydrogen on carbon 6 of the uracil in Figure 5, and so on, with this facility increasing in the order: alpha hydrogen greater than beta hydrogen.

In those molecules where the acidity allows these conditions to occur, both ketone and enolic forms can coexist, forming a dynamic chemical equilibrium. That is to say, one of these forms will pass to the other only by a change in the degree of acidity.

We can say that the energy contribution of the form on the right in Figure 1 can in some cases be up to 50% of that on the left, which means that it is possible that both ketone and enolic electronic forms can coexist independently, forming two distinct compounds, i.e. a ketone in equilibrium with its alcohol.

When defining the concept of pH, an important classification of ionic reactions in organic molecules is based on the nature of the reactive particle, which is conveniently assumed to be the attacking species. From that point of view, or according to the Gilbert Newton Lewis definition, the Lewis acid A in Figure 2 will be that species capable of accepting an electron pair; hence, its electronic charge is positive. Whereas a Lewis base B is the substance that gives up a pair of electrons; its electronic charge is negative.

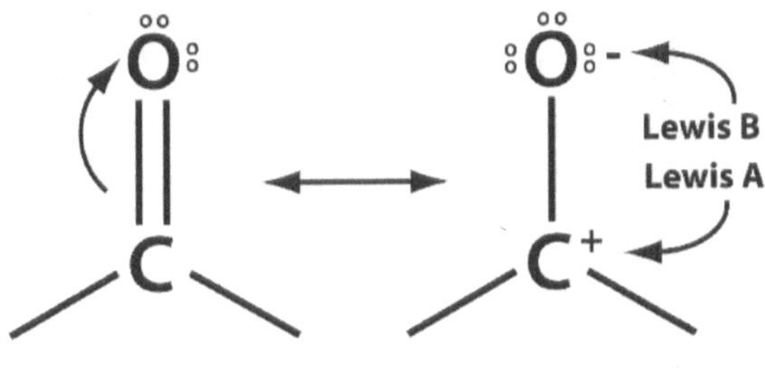

FIGURE 2

BEHAVIOUR OF THE CARBONYL GROUP AS A LEWIS A ACID, AND AS A LEWIS B BASE AT THE SAME TIME

With this definition established, we have that: those organic substances that are electron acceptors are called Lewis A acids, and are identified as electrophilic substances; that is, electrophilic species are those substances that have an affinity for particles that have an excess negative charge. Meanwhile, the electron donors are the Lewis B bases, and are called nucleophiles, since they are electron particles that have an affinity for nuclei, or those that carry a negative charge.

In this way, organic reactions are generated, which are classified as electrophilic and/or nucleophilic, depending on the type of electron-giving or electron-accepting reagent that gives rise to these reactions.

Therefore, we deduce that the carbonyl group of a ketone from which the conditions can be given for equilibrium to be formed with its alcohol, will behave simultaneously in the same molecule as a Lewis A acid, but at the same time, as a Lewis B base or alkali, such as the forms shown in Figure 2.

This is an inherent property or characteristic of the behaviour of the carbonyl group of a ketone having an alpha hydrogen, since the electrons tremolate from one form to the other in compounds where such a possibility exists, or, depending on the degree of acidity. This means that these substances will behave as Lewis A acids or Lewis B alkalis, and are subject to the acidic conditions of the medium in which they are immersed. Substances that have these characteristics of behaving as acids and bases depending on the degree of acidity are called amphoteric.

Thus, if the substance behaves as a base, it will pick up a Lewis A acid, as is the case with the bases guanine ketone and uracil, which can pick up a proton (H^+) in their carbonyl group from the acidic medium if they are behaving as ketones, or when the environment of the cell nucleus becomes acidic. In this case, it is the internal fluid of the cells affected by acidosis; this will influence the acidic conditions of the antioxidant system within the cells. Mainly NADH and NAD^+; which, as we have seen, is responsible for oxidising iron II in haemoglobin to iron III, and reducing iron III back to iron II, so that haemoglobin can transport oxygen as iron II and carbonic acid as iron III. In turn, the antioxidant system within the cells is needed to keep this range of acidity within its normal functionality.

If these high acidic conditions occur inside the cells, the carbonyl group of the ketone $=C=O$ will be transformed into an alcoholic group, $\equiv C-OH$. So, if the intercellular medium becomes acidic, the ketone, or Lewis base B in Figure 2, will be transformed into an alcohol; that is, a Lewis acid A. This is more stable and reactive than the ketone when the medium becomes more acidic.

Given these circumstances, this would force molecules where this situation is present to undergo electronic regrouping in the chromosomes in the nucleus, as happens to a ketone, or which was forced to transform into an alcohol. More stable enolate ions can form, such as those shown on the right of Figure 3.

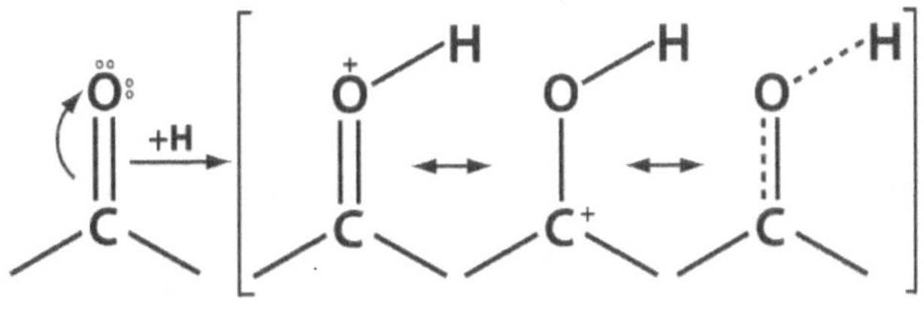

FIGURE 3

FORMATION OF AN ENOLATE ION FROM LEWIS ACID A ON THE CARBONYL GROUP OF A KETONE

If the process is reversed, on the enolate ion on the right in Figure 3, protonation takes place on the carbon, and the ketone will regenerate again. That would be what reverses the cancer. But if protonation occurs on oxygen, an enol ($\equiv$C-OH) will be formed. So, as can be seen in Figure 4, a C ketone with these changing characteristics, or one that has an alpha HA hydrogen, will be in equilibrium with its enol E, which will depend on the acidic conditions in the cell nucleus.

However, we can see that intermediate states can exist, as can be seen in Figure 3. Then, the Lewis acid A will be relatively less acidic, i.e. it will be a more basic acid.

The acidity moves on a relative scale between 0 and 14. When the acidity is between 0 and 7 it is considered acidic;

and from 7 to 14 it is said to be basic. It is assumed that at pH 7.00 the degree of acidity is neutral, although this point is difficult to achieve, since pH 7.00 is really a transitional state between acidity and alkalinity. A pH value equal to 7.00 is metastable.

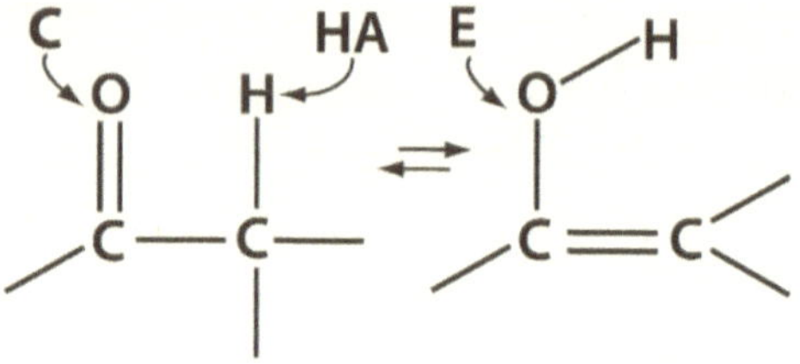

FIGURE 4

KETO-ENOLIC EQUILIBRIUM BETWEEN A KETONE C WITH ITS ALCOHOL AND THE ALPHA ALCOHOL AND THE ALPHA-HYDROGEN HA THAT CAN LEAVE TO FORM THE ENOL E

An important feature is that the ketone and enolic forms are real molecules. That is, they are separate and distinct substances and should not be confused with resonance isomers, which are only theoretical, highly reactive intermediate forms that do not stop to form stable substances or have a real physical existence. Whereas, it is possible to prepare enolates in the laboratory, as shown in Figures 3 and 4. That is why, in order to identify or describe the relationship between the ketone and enolic forms, another name has had to be adopted: they are called tautomers; and where these inter-conversions from keto- to enolic or from one form to the other occur, the phenomenon is known as tautomerism. Tautomer is derived from the English word taut.

At equilibrium, tautomers are formed; however, they quickly switch from one form to the other even under ordinary conditions. This is why it is difficult to isolate them for characterisation in the laboratory.

For the same reason, it is likely to be impossible from a practical point of view to measure this keto-enolic balance in the blood of a person suffering from cancer. At least in order to be able to prove that this is the cause of the cancer, or to prove the existence of these ketone and enolic compounds as two distinct and independent substances. Or, if you like, to explain the phenomenon of tautomerism, which is evident and reasonable from the point of view deduced by electronic and theoretical analysis of the molecular structure of each molecule that is likely to participate in a tautomerism process. We owe the concept of tautomerism to the Dutch chemist Jacobus Henricus van 't Hoff.

Since it is impossible to measure, for example, the degree of displacement of the tautomeric equilibrium of a DNA in vivo, attempts have been made to simulate this equilibrium by in vitro experiments using the so-called "Combined Density Functional Theory" with the Poisson-Boltzmann continuous solution model. This is a quantum theoretical method, which will only lead to a theoretical probability by experimental simulation. However, tautomerism can be deduced theoretically, just by sharpening the analysis, and knowing the chemical characteristics of the five bases that make up the DNA and RNA of cells, such as the bases that make up DNA shown in Figure 5.

In Figure 5 we can distinguish the five bases that are in the nucleus of cells for chromosomes to build the DNA sequence and ribosomes to build proteins. The four bases involved in forming DNA are: adenine A, guanine G, thymine T and cytosine C. The linking groups that are not shown are the dashed bar lines (---) that correspond to the deoxyribose sugar molecules that form the side chains of DNA, or what we have already identified as nucleosides. The uracil base does not participate in the conformation of DNA; the uracil base only participates in the conformation of RNA.

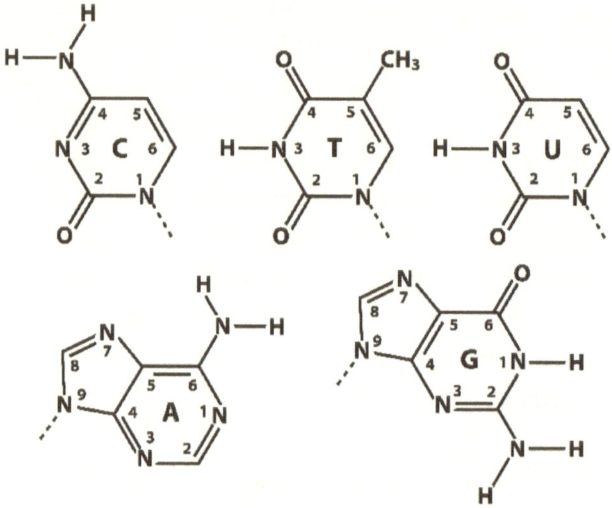

FIGURE 5

THE FIVE BASES THAT ARE AT THE CORE OF A HEALTHY CELL HEALTHY CELL

These bases are formed in the nucleus from folate; and folinic acid is formed from folate. Folate is found in green fruits; and one of the active forms of folate is folic acid, which is why its consumption is recommended during pregnancy to prevent genetic errors in the foetus, such as bifid or open spines.

Under the strictest conditions of acidity or the normal chemical environment inside the nucleus of cells, in chromosomes, the thymine base is achieved by participating only in DNA; but the thymine base does not participate in the formation of RNA.

It means that, somehow in the nucleus of cells, the bases that make up DNA are prone to changes, which occur according to the acidic or basic conditions of the nucleus. It is this that determines the shape of these original base-pair couplings in the chromosomes. Therefore, the acid-base conditions for the couplings to occur will be determined by the degree of acidity that prevails within the nucleus of the cells; because, as you can see, this very specific form of base pairing depends on the functions that each base pair must fulfil in the DNA and RNA inside and outside the nucleus.

If we look at Figure 5, we notice that the only thing that differentiates the thymine base from the uracil base is that the thymine base has the methyl group ($-CH_3$) inserted on carbon 5 of the ring. Somehow, either because the methyl group is a reactive negative charge-giving species, this methyl group is close to the ketone group of thymine, which does not allow the thymine base to tautomerise, or the ketone thymine base to become an enol.

The other reason is that, at carbon 5, the methyl group replaced the alpha hydrogen, so thymine cannot undergo tautomerism. The thymine base only has a beta hydrogen at carbon 6, but the thymine base is less likely to be tautomerised. Whereas, relatively speaking, or from a probability point of view, tautomerism will occur more strongly in the ketonic guanine base, because the oxygen in the ketonic guanine will attract the proton from the acidic medium, or from the nitrogen that is adjacent to the ketone group, i.e. nitrogen number 1, as shown in Figure 5.

As for the uracil base, we can see in Figure 5, that the uracil base has two alpha hydrogens adjacent to the carbonyl group on carbon number 4; specifically on nitrogen number 3 and carbon number 5. Thus, a double bond can be formed in uracil as soon as the uracil is transformed from the ketonic form to an enol by the hydrogen leaving carbon number 5. Then, the alpha hydrogen on the number 3 nitrogen will come out more easily, which is more likely to happen on the enolic uracil base. Thus, when the medium is acidic, methylation will occur to the enolic uracil base, as shown in Figure 12.

The bases adenine and guanine are those that correspond to the purine group, i.e. these are less basic bases. The bases cytosine, thymine and uracil belong to the pyrimidine group, i.e. they are more basic bases.

According to what we have seen in this keto-enolic equilibrium, those bases that contain in their electronic structure ketone groups (=C=O), plus an alpha hydrogen that can be detached, these bases can be configured in the form of an enol, that is, an alcohol ($\equiv$C-OH) so that a double bond is produced in the ring. Thus, this base will become a more aromatically stable molecule when the chemical environment becomes acidic.

Whereas, the cytosine base, despite having a ketone group on carbon 2, this pyrimidine base has the electronic characteristic of not having an alpha hydrogen on the adjacent nitrogen on carbon number 1 and 3 of its ketone group. In other words, cytosine does not have an alpha hydrogen that can be detached to capture one of the bonds and then stably close the ring, which is a necessary condition for the enol to form. The double bond in the ring of the cytosine base is complete with hydrogen atoms, so that the cytosine base is unalterable for an electronic tautomerism process to occur.

We conclude that what can happen to the cytosine base is methylation when the cellular environment becomes more acidic, as the high acidity will expose carbon 5 of the cytosine ring to nucleophiles or nucleosome scavenging groups such as the methyl radical ($\cdot$CH$_3$) when the cellular environment becomes more acidic. Or when such methyl groups are more abundant due to the consumption of animal protein.

This leads to demethylation of the amino acid methionine. The amino acid methionine is the one most frequently found in all animal proteins, because the amino acid methionine is the one that marks the initiation triplet for the ribosome; in other words, methionine is the code that tells the ribosome to 'start here', so that the ribosome can begin the process of making a protein. So, methionine comes in all animal proteins.

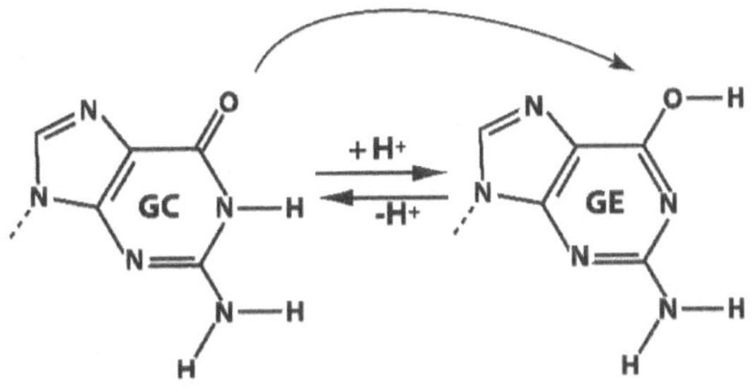

FIGURE 6

TAUTOMERISM IN GUANINE: IF THE MEDIUM IS ACIDIC KETONIC GUANINE GC WILL CONVERT TO ENOLIC GUANINE GE

The correct coupling or not of these two bases depends on the modification that the chromosomes must make to change the electronic structure of the DNA. For, in normal DNA, the bases are electronically bonded by hydrogen bonds (the dotted line in Figure 8; H---O=C=, H---N=). The bonds or bridges that form between the hydrogen atoms are known as Van der Waals Forces.

As we will see in more detail in the case of methylation, this change occurs because the consumption of the meat of another animal brings the cells, proteins and cholesterol that is specific to each animal lineage, which is why heart attacks occur. The protein in animal meat is rich in the amino acid methionine, which causes methylation and induces cancer.

The amino acid methionine, on losing its methyl group, will become homocysteine; which, as well as leaving us with an abundance of the methyl group, will cause the bases cytosine and uracil to both convert to thymine. The amino acid homocysteine is also an antioxidant agent; therefore, homocysteine will usurp the antioxidant role of the other natural antioxidants inside the cells, such as: the enzyme superoxide dismutase, alkaline phosphatase, hexokinase and oxidised NAD^+ and reduced NADH, which, as we have seen, have the function of modifying the iron oxidation state of haemoglobin. So, that haemoglobin alternately transports oxygen and carbon dioxide in the form of carbonic acid.

We do not need to consume proteins to live, but the amino acids that these chains contain, which we can find in a more abundant and varied way in vegetables. As we said, the enzyme pepsin in the stomach will break down these proteins to obtain the amino acids. For example, in rice and legumes, the proteins are shorter chain, so they are easier to digest than animal meat protein. However, these proteins from legumes and rice are not complete, i.e. these proteins do not contain all the essential amino acids. The protein of meat, for example beef, is complete, because the cow obtained its full ration of essential and non-essential amino acids only by eating various kinds of vegetables. But by eating rice with legumes, we get a large part of the 8 essential amino acids from this combination.

In fact, vegetarian animals such as hippopotamuses, gorillas, cows, giraffes and elephants eat only vegetables to get their daily ration of amino acids. Humans do not need to kill other beings to eat them, because food is most abundantly found in vegetables, but we will not have to run after an animal to kill it. The domestication of animals, in the misnamed animal agriculture, is a deception towards our brothers, who are the ones who pay with their misfortune for this ignorance of human food.

Chapter 3

COUPLING BETWEEN THE BASES

In normal DNA, the ketonic guanine base can form hydrogen bonds with the hydrogen bonded to nitrogen atom 1 and with the hydrogen of the nitrogen of the amino group, which is bonded to carbon number 2, as can be seen in Figure 5. Of the three pyrimidinic bases such as thymine, uracil and cytosine in the nucleus that can meet this condition of coupling with the ketonic guanine base, it is the cytosine base.

There is no other pyrimidine base that has the same electronic characteristics but the cytosine base. Moreover, this coupling is achieved by both bases in a conjugated form. As can be seen in Figure 7, which shows how the guanine ketone base contributes to hydrogen bonding via the amino group attached to carbon number 2. Additionally, they are joined by the hydrogen atom that is bonded to their number 1 nitrogen. Meanwhile, the cytosine base contributes to the formation of the hydrogen bond, also from its amino group that is bonded to carbon number 4.

This triple bond strength is reciprocal; therefore, this is the most stable form of coupling that forms DNA. Whereas, this chemical condition with the ketonic guanine base cannot be fulfilled by the uracil base. Therefore, the uracil base cannot bind to the ketonic guanine base or the adenine base to form DNA. We conclude that, naturally or normally, in DNA, the ketonic guanine base can only form hydrogen bonds with the cytosine base, as there is no other base that can form this bond.

The adenine base has only two possibilities, as it has a single hydrogen in its amino group attached to its number 6 carbon. So, in order for the adenine base to form a hydrogen bond with an oxygen, this coupling can only be achieved if adenine accepts a hydrogen bond at its number 1 nitrogen in order to form two hydrogen bonds. This is a chemical condition that is only possible between the base adenine and the base thymine. In such a case, and as we can see in Figure 5, the adenine base could couple with the uracil ketone base; but, this is only in a relative way, because the thymine base is more basic than the uracil base. Since the thymine base, as we said, carries on carbon number 5 of its ring the methyl group which replaced the alpha hydrogen. Thus, this methyl group gives the thymine base greater energetic stability.

From an electronic point of view, the uracil base will not be able to couple with the adenine base either. But there is no other base in the cell nucleus that performs with the same or similar electronic characteristics as the thymine base, or another base that could fulfil this condition to replace it.

So, the uracil base does not fit with the adenine base or the ketonic guanine base to form hydrogen bonds; as long as the acidic condition within the nucleus is normal, for DNA to replicate in that specific way under standard DNA acidity conditions. Because if this did not happen in this way, the two ketone groups of the thymine base would face each other in one row of the DNA side chain; and these ketone groups would repel or reject each other, breaking the sequence on that side of the helix in the DNA chain.

In the normal DNA or N-DNA shown in Figure 10, we see that another hydrogen bond forms between the thymine and cytokine bases. This bond makes the DNA strand twist like a spiral. The thymine-cytokine bond is lost in the event of cancer.

Thus, neither the uracil base nor the thymine base can couple with the ketonic guanine base to form a chain structure in normal DNA. Whereas, this chemical structure for coupling can only be fulfilled by the cytosine base with the ketonic guanine base.

Cancer is a chemical phenomenon, so we need to know what these couplings are like to know how cancer can be generated chemically, because the DNA that gives each cell its structure is made up of electronic matter, which will make the necessary adjustments between the electronic couplings. Compound cells were formed by the mutation of viruses; therefore, cells are not aware of their existence or their performance in living beings, even though they are only chemically functional beings.

Furthermore, the form of these base-to-base couplings is electronic matter that was formed from electronic energy. So, it, and all forms of matter, can be expected to change constantly, because it can form an infinite number of kinds and combinations among the infinite ranges of energy and different kinds of matter of electronic origin.

Whereas the spirit is only made up of magnetic mass, and may or may not be aware of the mechanism of the coupling of the bases in the DNA of the cells that make up its physical body, which is made up of electronic matter. It is only the knowledge of the spirit that will be aware of how these couplings occur, and knowledge is gained through learning.

The cells of a living body have no memory; for these cells come from a diploid. The diploid comes from the integration of two haploids: one haploid comes from the gonads of the male and the other haploid comes from the egg of the female. Memory is brought by the spirit in magnetic form, which is incorporated into the baby in the womb, 5 months after gestation when the diploid has become a baby with her or his sex defined.

The spirit and the body are two different kinds of energies. The physical body contains only electronic matter; whereas, the spirit inhabiting the physical body is made up of magnetic mass without electronic matter.

The physical world is only a station for the spatial attraction between the female and the male gender. In the human race, these two magnetic and electronic energies form the energies of a woman and a man. The female comes from the integration of negative fermions, and the male from the integration of positive fermions. But this physical attraction is the same for all genders of living organisms.

What is defined as death on earth cannot exist in any form, for it is impossible for the electronic matter of the physical body to die, and the probability of the magnetic mass of the spirit dying is nil. There is only a separation of the two kinds of energy. The magnetic mass separates from the electronic matter of the body when the electronic body completes its physical changes in its evolutionary state. On Earth this is called old age. It is only a moment; for, time does not exist in the spiritual world. At that moment of disconnection, the electronic matter of the body will be devoid of the magnetic mass that gave it life, and the evolving electronic matter of the body will be free on Earth; thus, it will continue to change with the passing of time. Whereas the magnetic mass of the spirit will be eternally magnetic mass in the eternal moment. What the magnetic mass of the spirit gains at birth is the knowledge during the time it was part of a physical body.

This phenomenon of the coupling between the bases in the DNA is the result of the combination of these two kinds of energies by a condition which we now say is chemical in nature. This is vital for the manifestation of physical life through the correct coupling of the bases in DNA. For the electronic matter forms a sequence of couplings, which give the physical characteristics to each individual by means of a genetic code.

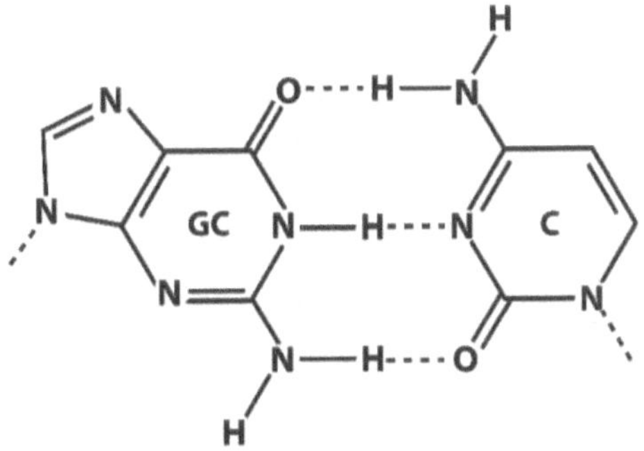

FIGURE 7

HYDROGEN BRIDGING OF KETONIC GUANINE GC COUPLED TO CYTOSINE C BASE IN NORMAL DNA

For this integration of the two kinds of energy to have that functionality or life form, the purine bases can be coupled with the pyrimidine bases in a specific way, or only in that way: the ketonic guanine base coupled with the cytosine base, and the adenine base will bind only with the thymine base. Since the uracil base does not meet these conditions, the uracil base cannot participate in or be part of DNA, as shown in Figure 8.

The four bases will pair up in DNA via hydrogen bonds, forming pairs or groups of two, which will be paired in the way we have already mentioned: the pair formed by the adenine=thymine bases, and the pair formed by the guanine-keto ≡cytosine bases joined by two and three hydrogen bonds respectively. But, in normal DNA, another hydrogen bridge is formed between the two pyrimidine base pairs; that is, the thymine-cytosine hydrogen bridge.

In this case, these base pairs cause the two nucleotide chains that make up DNA to be joined by the hydrogen bridges represented by the dotted lines between the bases formed by three base pairs: adenine-thymine, thymine-cytosine and guanine ketone-cytosine.

So, the junction in this stretch of DNA, as we can see, is actually more complex than the simple junction between the bases adenine=thymine (A=T), thymine-cytokine (T-C) and guanine≡cytosine (G≡C). This makes DNA both crammed together and twisted together as the most fascinating molecule known in life-forming chemistry.

At the lateral ends of the DNA molecule, nucleotide bonds are formed between the nucleotides by ligands with the sugar molecules deoxyribose and phosphoric acid. These bonds create a left-to-right twisting effect of the DNA. For the left-to-right twist of this spiral, all the deoxyribose molecules must be right-handed, but in sequential order. Therefore, a left-handed sugar cannot intervene with a right-handed sugar, because it would be a huge mess; or there would be no life.

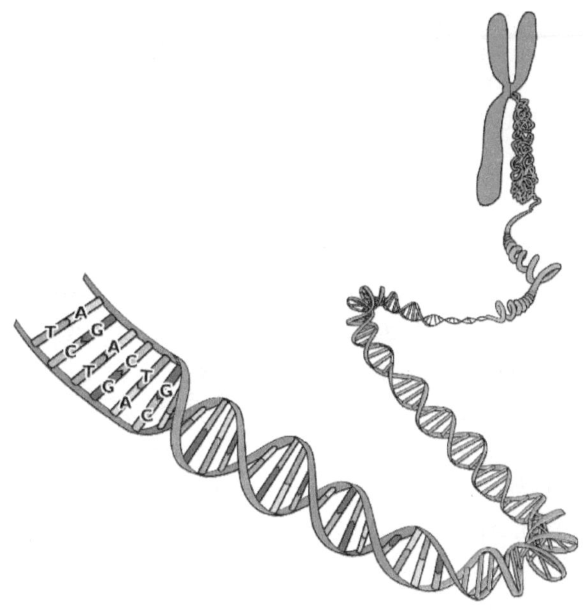

FIGURE 8

A DNA MOLECULE SYNTHESISED BY CHROMOSOMES. IT IS THE MOST EXTRAORDINARY MOLECULE IN CHEMISTRY; BECAUSE IT IS THE ELECTRONIC MOLECULE THAT GIVES THE ENERGY OF LIFE TO ALL BEINGS ON EARTH

The same is true for protein formation: all amino acids involved in protein formation are left-handed, but there is no sequence of left-handed and right-handed amino acids. Right-handed amino acids are not involved in protein conformation; because a sequence of left-handed and right-handed amino acids would not allow proteins to roll up three-dimensionally. If it were a left-handed amino acid followed by a right-handed amino acid, proteins would be straight and physical bodies would not exist. Proteins have to be three-dimensional, because among other functions, these molecules form the filling of the skeleton of the physical body.

This form of coupling between left-handed and right-handed molecules is due to chirality; just as the chirality of amino acids makes proteins, where all the amino acids involved in proteins are left-handed; and when you try to introduce a right-handed amino acid, it will not fit because it would change the sequence of amino acids in the protein chain.

The bonds of these rungs are due to both chirality and the strength of the hydrogen bonds between the pairs of the purine bases adenine and guanine with the pyrimidine bases thymine and cytosine. Whereas, the continuous lateral lines linking these pairs are formed by the coupling of these two base pairs. Therefore, we have said that acidity or basicity are relative terms, since other electronic bonding forces, such as hydrogen bonds, are involved in joining the atoms.

As indicated, the phenomenon of tautomerism can only happen to the ketonic guanine bases, and to uracil when the uracil has become enolic. This happens as soon as the chemical environment of the cell nucleus becomes more acidic. When this happens, the ketone group on the number 6 carbon of the guanine base, or the number 4 of the uracil, will make the ketonic guanine and uracil bases enolic. In other words, guanine and uracil in alcoholic form became a form of bases which, instead of giving, now accept electronic charges in order to form hydrogen bonds. We can say that when the guanine and uracil bases were ketonic, that made them nucleophilic bases, or Lewis bases. But logically, when acidity is high in the cell nucleus, the ketonic guanine and uracil bases become enolic bases; that is, they are now electrophilic, or Lewis acids.

Whereas the alpha hydrogens, i.e. the number 1 of the ketonic guanine and the number 5 and 3 of the uracil, being weak bonds, these hydrogens may be prone to leave easily, when a change of acidity to a higher value occurs. Thus, the hydrogen of the amino group on carbon number 2 of the enolic guanine base ring will remain an acceptor of electronic charges. When the uracil base becomes enolic, it loses the hydrogen on nitrogen 3; thus, a hydrogen bridge can no longer form at that site.

This amino group on the enolic guanine will continue to form the hydrogen bridge, as we can see in Figure 9 for the case of the enolic guanine. Therefore, the nitrogen number 1 of the enolic guanine base is now depleted of hydrogen, which means that the enolic guanine base can no longer form a hydrogen bridge specifically at this site, i.e. there is no longer any alpha hydrogen in the enolic guanine base that can be released to form a double bond.

However, the guanine base with its enolic form will be able to form a hydrogen bridge with the nitrogen atom which has lost its alpha hydrogen. But the only base that can provide the hydrogen to form such a hydrogen bond is the thymine base, i.e. base number 2 in Figure 5. Since, due to tautomerism, the uracil base became similar to the cytosine base, it does not have a hydrogen on its nitrogen number 3, as can be seen in Figure 5.

Therefore, this new and circumstantial requirement cannot be fulfilled by the cytosine bases, nor by the uracil, but by the thymine base in its ketonic form, as soon as the ketonic guanine base and the uracil base become bases with an enolic electronic configuration. So, to form a coupling with the guanine base in its enolic form, the only base left in the nucleus of the cells for the chromosomes to form the hydrogen bond as in Figure 8, is the thymine base.

If we look again at Figure 5, perhaps this requirement can be better fulfilled by the thymine base with the enolic guanine base, because in this case of a higher acidity, the ketone group on carbon number 4 of the thymine base has to be more stabilised. Because the thymine base has a methyl group on carbon number 5 of its ring and no alpha hydrogen, the thymine base is resistant to tautomerism, but this stability is thanks to the contribution of the methyl group on carbon number 5 of the thymine base in Figure 5.

Acidosis and methylation cause the uracil base and the cytochrome base to be lost from the cell nucleus. Because these two bases will be converted to thymine when tautomerism occurs in the cytosine and uracil enol bases. Ultimately, it is the thymine base in DNA that can make up for this lack of cytosine and uracil, because it is the only base that can couple with the enolic guanine base, as can be seen in Figure 10.

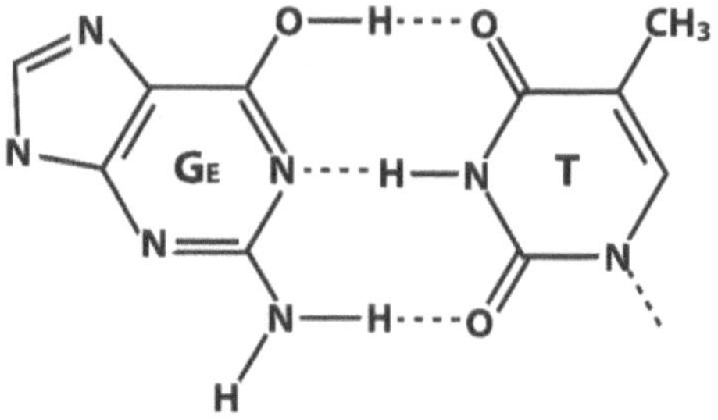

FIGURE 9

IN DNA, GUANINE IN THE ENOLIC FORM GE CAN ONLY COUPLE WITH THE THYMINE BASE

Looking at what Figures 3 and 6 show regarding tautomerism in the uracil and guanine bases, let's look at Figure 10 to see what happens when the guanine base is transformed from its ketonic form to the enolic spatial configuration in the cell's DNA, which is a relatively more stable electronic condition under these conditions of acidosis.

Now, however, conditions have arisen so that instead of being with the cytosine base, the coupling of the guanine base to its enolic form occurs with the thymine base. As shown in Figure 9.

This increase in acidity, as we have said, originated from the acidic condition of the cytoplasm and then in the nucleus; which, in turn, was caused by excess uric acid, carbonic acid and lactic acid, as a product of haemolysis and glycolysis in the mitochondria of muscle cells. Since the process of respiration was affected, and the supply of oxygen by the normal route of respiration decreased. This, in turn, affected the oxidation/anti-oxidation system, and so on. Thereafter, the enzyme complex, which before acidosis was controlled by the cell itself, will be disrupted.

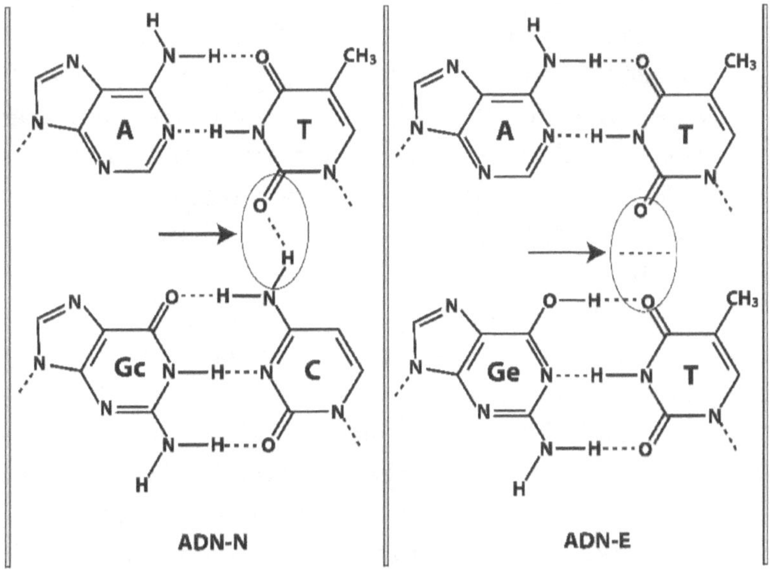

FIGURE 10

N-DNA: NORMAL DNA KETONIC GUANIN Gc COUPLED WITH CYTOSIN. E-DNA: ENOLIC GUANINE Ge COUPLED WITH THE THYMININE BASE. THIS IS HOW THE DNA MUTATION THAT GIVES RISE TO CANCER ORIGINS.

This adverse condition started, as we have shown, by the imbalance of concentrations between uric acid and sodium urate: [uric acid] $\leftrightarrow$ [sodium urate] [H$^+$ protons], from the moment we started to ingest the inactive animal meat cells. Since, as we saw, we need the concentration of our antioxidant sodium urate to be at least 40 times higher than the concentration of uric acid.

So, cells carrying this erroneous DNA AND-E in Figure 10, lose their structure or electronic configuration, as well as their original chemical property, and problems related to this distorted gene sequence can occur.

Replication of these mutant cells induces, for example, a slight tumour, which, as it progresses in size, will become visible as a cancer as the replication of these genetically active cells proceeds. However, despite being active, these cells replicate faster than healthy cells. They are changeable, because that is the nature of the electronic matter that forms DNA to seek its electronic readjustment, depending on the acidic conditions for the chromosomes within the cell nucleus, as shown in Figure 10.

So, by causing acidosis, we have also succeeded in changing the ketonic or normal molecular structure of ketonic guanine and uracil. Therefore, the conditions necessary for the natural formation of hydrogen bonds (H---O=C=, H---N=) will also be changed. Because in any case, the tautomeric or enolic structure of the guanine can only couple with the ketonic or normal structure of the thymine base, thus introducing a coupling error into the mutated DNA.

The triple bond that the guanine base has to form with the cytosine base must possess the particular characteristic of contributing its fifth hydrogen bond between the thymine and cytosine base pairs, which, as mentioned, confers greater energetic stability and three-dimensionality to the DNA, which strengthens or stabilises the original DNA structure. Therefore, this influence as a triple bond must be important. As a fifth thymine-cytosine bridge, it must also give the DNA greater stability, as can be seen on the left of Figure 10. That is, hydrogen bridge number 3. These hydrogen bonds produce a crowding, which imposes a high energy stability on the normal DNA.

Whereas, this hydrogen bridge between the thymine base and the cytokine base disappears when the guanine base in enolic form couples with the thymine base. That is, the hydrogen bridge between the base pairs is gone, as shown by the dashed line in Figure 10. So, the strength of the triple bond is less in the wrong DNA, and in a way, the wrong DNA becomes energetically weaker. Less energy will be needed to synthesise the mismatched DNA, and the mutated DNA will replicate faster than the normal DNA, as in the case of cancer.

It is a transition type mutation, because it is caused by substitution between bases of the same class, i.e. pyrimidine for pyrimidine, (the base cytosine for the base thymine) which is more likely, as this form of coupling does not introduce a substantial change in the normal chemical structure, or that of the original DNA, as can be seen in Figure 9.

However, the chromosomes of a cell that are involved in this tautomerism, and if the tautomerism becomes peremptory, the cell will be able to continue with its reproductive work, but, routed by a logic of chemical character of its chromosomes, as can be seen in Figure 8.

DNA synthesis will be at odds with other cells, at least in terms of speed of replication and functionality. This cell will not be fit to configure the electronic matter of the body of a human being born with a conglomerate of normal cells. But, a change in the structure of their genes was introduced by their way of feeding. Therefore, these mutant cells belonging to the same body will come into conflict with the other healthy cells.

It is important to know, as we have said, that these differences are relative to each other, because in the electronic bonds there does not necessarily have to be a marked contrast for the necessary adjustments to take place and for the couplings between the bases to be conducive. In a relative sense, it can be said that if there were to be an abundance of methyl groups within the cell nucleus, the cytosine base would no longer be available, because in the methylation process, as we shall see, the entire cytosine base would be converted to the thymine base, which is the partner of the adenine base.

So, that cell nucleus, when it is involved in a tautomerism and methylation process, will energetically transform into a relatively stable and functional chemical configuration, under those conditions of higher acidity in the cell nucleus, so that the chromosomes in Figure 8 replicate the DNA in the wrong way. But their rate of replication, while logical from a chemical point of view, will be altered from a biological perspective, and that is what shows up in what we call a mutation. It is no longer the same molecule of the original DNA that developed in the same body made of electronic matter and magnetic mass.

It is not a condition that can be inherited by genetic modification in all cells, because such a change in the already formed genes would be complicated to happen in the same body. A person in the terminal stage of cancer cannot give birth to a mutated being, or one that carries the mutation with it; or a pregnant woman who has acquired her pregnancy during the formation of mutant cells can pass on distorted DNA to the foetus, so the child may suffer from cancer inherited from the mother. If this were the case, we would conclude that cancer could not be reversed in children born with the mutated cells, but we know that the mutation can be reversed in a person born without cancer.

It is an error in the coupling caused by acidosis that alters the bond between the bases that make up DNA, which is possible to restore chemically, because healthy cells are developing in a design pattern, which is determined by the traits of the genes.

It is different if we are born with a DNA that has one or several altered genes, or which already have a modified or implicit DNA structure; because this modification only has to be provided by the male haploid with half of its chromosomes, and the other half of chromosomes that come from the female haploid represented by the ovum. For this to happen, one of the two pairs of chromosomes must already be modified. In other words, if the cancer were inherited, the genetic error could come from either the father or the mother.

It is also possible to change the configuration of the poly anion of the phosphate groups; and the complex formed by the reducing enzymes, whose main representatives are: glutathioneSH, hexokinase, catalase, superoxide dismutase, active vitamin C, etc., and which were the ones that protected the DNA against changes in relative acidity inside the cell. In other words, the chemical and energetic circumstances are right for the bonds to form between the enolic guanine-thymine base pairs instead of being ketonic guanine-cytosine, and so the cancer or mutation in the cell arises.

The shape of the couplings must have happened for a very specific reason. It could be, for example, the increased speed at which each different organism needs to read its codes in order to synthesise, for example, at a faster rate a particular protein by its ribosomes. Or a higher frequency of replication of their DNA in their chromosomes. So, each organism will have its own moment of life, which will depend on the speed with which its cells replicate. This will have an influence, because it is what determines the culmination of the ageing of each race of living beings.

We might think that the first humans did not eat meat. Uracil was present only in RNA, for the purpose of speeding up protein synthesis in ribosomes. But it was not in the DNA, because if it had been, the replication of the DNA in the chromosomes in Figure 8 would have happened in a more hurried manner. Likewise, if the thymine base were in RNA, protein synthesis would have happened too slowly. In other words, there would be no life.

In April 1997 an article appeared in the Proceedings of the National Academy of Sciences of the United States of America PNAS (PNAS April 1, 1997, vol. 94no. 73290-3295) by researchers Benjamin C. Blount et al. entitled: "Folate deficiency causes incorrect incorporation of uracil into human DNA and chromosome breakage, with implications for cancer and neural damage". This is what we call open spines in the case of folic acid. The spine is also known as the vertebral column, because the cervical vertebrae generally have a forked "Y" shape. Perhaps the most important thing about this article, in this specific case, is that these researchers were able to demonstrate experimentally that the uracil base, which should only be in the various RNAs, was mistakenly introduced into the DNA. But these thymine and enolic uracil bases are virtually identical, so we won't know whether it is the thymine base that actually causes the DNA breakage in a person with cancer, or whether it is the thymine base when it is coupled into the DNA with the guanine base in enolic form.

Chapter 4

METHYLATION

Methylation is necessary to introduce the methyl group ($\cdot CH_3$) into molecules. Mainly in amino acids that carry this methyl group, such as aromatic amino acids, which cannot be produced by animals, so these amino acids are called essential amino acids. An example of an amino acid that carries a methyl group is methionine. Essential amino acids are only made by plants.

Consumption of protein from an animal source will create an excess of the amino acid methionine; in this case, the methyl group of the amino acid methionine can be detached; and, the methyl radical will be free. This radical is a nucleophile, and has a high reactivity, whose negative charge should be consumed on the inside of the cells by the antioxidant system, and by sodium urate and vitamin C on the outside of the cells.

However, if the cell nucleus or the blood becomes acidic, the methyl radical released from methionine cannot be neutralised. In this case, on the inside of the cells, the methyl radical will react with the cytosine and uracil bases in their enolic form, and convert both bases to the thymine base, as shown in Figures 11 and 12 respectively.

In the case of the cytosine base in Figure 11, when the methyl captures this cytosine base, it will be transformed into the thymine base. Similarly, the same happens to the uracil base, when uracil is in the enolic form as a result of high acidity; as can be seen in Figure 12. That is, the uracil base in the enolic form will be affected by a methylation process when the acidic environment converts the uracil base from its ketone form to its enolic form.

Eventually, or after this methylation process, the nucleus of that cell will be left without the bases cytosine and uracil, because both bases will be converted to thymine. So, in order to replicate DNA, the chromosomes will use the thymine base as a substitute for the cytosine base, which will now be in abundance in the nucleus of that cell.

So, if there were no acidosis in the cells, tautomerism in the guanine and uracil bases would not occur. If tautomerism did not occur, methylation of the cytosine and uracil bases would not occur.

It is the carnivorous lifestyle we are trying to adapt to, which will only result in our cells becoming cancerous units. It is a mutation, i.e. an electronic adaptation made by the chromosomes in the nucleus, according to the degree of acidity prevailing within the cells.

Generally speaking, all meat is harmful, because absolutely all meat comes from living beings; and therefore, all animals, as well as humans, are made up of cells; these cells are made up of DNA and RNA, which contain the purine bases guanine and adenine. Animal protein, on the other hand, contains an excess of the amino acid methionine, which, when it loses its methyl group, is converted into the amino acid homocysteine.

Methionine is a methyl group donor $-CH_3$; therefore, methionine can be considered as a product of homocysteine methylation. Thus, homocysteine is energetically more stable than methionine; therefore, if the acidity level is high, methionine can have its methyl group removed to become homocysteine. This methyl group detached from methionine will cause the cytosine and uracil bases to convert to the thymine base as mentioned above.

If there is tautomerism, the thymine base will be in abundance in the nucleus of the cell; and to make the couplings where the cytosine and uracil bases are missing, the chromosomes will use the thymine base to form DNA and RNA. But, that DNA will become mutant, because it will continue to replicate at a faster rate with this new wrong shape than the DNA and RNA of normal cells in the same body. In other words, the replication process of both the mutated DNA and RNA is accelerated, relative to the rate of replication of normal DNA and RNA.

However, we will only notice this abnormality when we observe that there is a lump or abnormal growth due to a tumour somewhere in the soft tissue of the body; since 80% of cancer cases occur in the epithelial membranes of organs. Specifically, in the apical cells of these epithelial membranes. Say, inside the milk ducts of the breast, the uterus, the seminal vesicles near the prostate, the liver, the pancreas, the lungs, the throat or in the epidermis. These are all soft tissues formed by apical epithelial cells. For example, the human beings who suffer most from cancer are women because of the involvement of the uterus, and in second place are men because of cancer in the seminal vesicles close to the prostate. Inhabitants of the Nordic countries are affected by skin cancer, because they are exposed to sunstroke in the tropics and the ultraviolet rays affect the apical cells of the epidermis.

While the lack of uracil in RNA, whose function has now been taken over by thymine, will lead to errors in protein synthesis by ribosomes on the outside of the nucleus, i.e. in the cytosol of the cell. This happens because the protein synthesis codes are already altered from the chromosomes to the ribosomes, and the ribosomes will not be able to read these synthesis codes. So, the protein sequence is altered, because the code implicit in the messenger RNA does not correspond to the code of the transfer RNA. So, the ribosomes are electronically disassembled and will synthesise a kind of protein that is not functional for normal human cells.

As it turns out, these now-mutant cells will replicate faster than healthy cells, because the energy force that stabilises the wrong DNA is lower. In other words, the time will come when there will be more mutant cells than normal cells. The mitochondria of the cells are affected to a lesser extent, because they are better able to adapt to the high acidity that occurs inside the cells.

However, if the degree of acidity on the outside of the cells, i.e. in the blood, is increased, the sodium urate will be completely transformed into free uric acid, specifically 3-methyluric acid, and we will lose the antioxidant sodium urate and vitamin C through urine and perspiration. With that, oxidative stress will start to get out of control; which will, for example, cause more of the methionine consumed from animal protein to be converted into homocysteine.

In the normal acidic condition, oxidative stress is necessary for the mechanism of haemolysis, or the breakdown of red blood cells that have ceased to perform their transport functions. At the same time, antioxidants help to prevent healthy red blood cells from prematurely losing their function of transporting oxygen and carbon dioxide alternately.

Inside the cells, when methionine is converted into homocysteine, homocysteine will usurp the function of the cells' own antioxidants. So, in this way, it will start to reduce the respiratory enzyme system, which, as we have seen, is important within cells to control the degree of acidity when generating energy in the form of heat without oxygen in the mitochondria.

Energy without oxygen is needed in cases of distress. For example, when we are frightened we stop breathing; and cortisol causes the insulin level to drop so that more glucose is available in case we have to make a run for it. The process of breathing without oxygen through glycolysis is most developed in birds, reptiles, insects and diving animals, such as turtles, seals and penguins. Diving animals have to dive into the water to search for food, but then they have to come to the surface to breathe oxygen from the air. But humans are not divers; humans only live on the surface of the Earth where they breathe in oxygen from the air.

As we have already explained, it is difficult for cytosine to be tautomerised, because its ring has complete double bonds. So, the cytosine base does not have an alpha hydrogen, or one that is adjacent to the ketone group on carbon number 2, in order to close another double bond between two carbon atoms in the cytosine base ring.

In other words, the most likely thing that can happen to the cytosine base is methylation, due to the weakening produced by the higher degree of acidity on the amino group attached to carbon 4 of the cytosine base ring.

The higher acidity, as we saw, is the result of glycolysis, or the fermentation of glucose; that is, the process of cellular respiration without oxygen; since, by this route of glycolysis or fermentation of glucose, lactic acid will be generated in the mitochondria. Mainly in the muscle cells, which are the cells that need to produce more energy, because they are in motion; in addition, muscle cells are more abundant in the body.

If oxygen does not reach these cells, the mitochondria will resort to producing caloric energy through glycolysis.

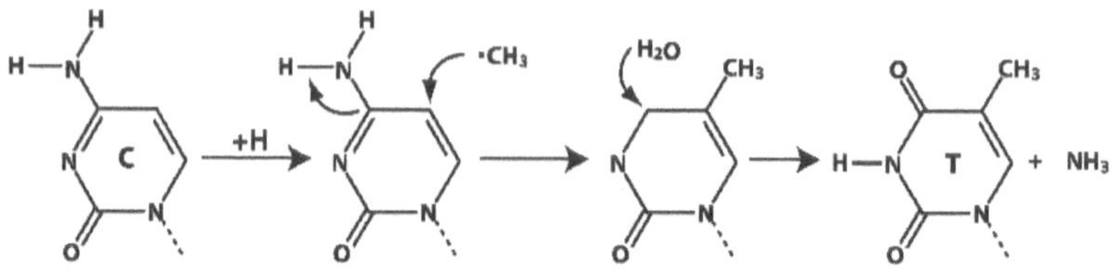

FIGURE 11

CONVERSION OF THE CYTOSINE C BASE TO THE THYMINE T BASE BY METHYLATION

On the other hand, as cytosine becomes acidic, carbon 5 in the cytosine ring will become positive, i.e., electrophile, and vulnerable to attack by free radicals or nucleophiles, such as the methyl group ($\cdot CH_3$). Which, being an electron giving group. This methyl group can react with nuclei; that is, with those particles that have a positive charge, as shown by the curved arrows in Figure 11.

In the case of Figure 11 for the cytosine base, the methyl radical ($\cdot CH_3$) left over from the methionine will attack carbon 5 on the cytosine ring, and this will convert it into an intermediate, i.e. 5-methylcytosine. Then, as the 5-methylcytosine compound loses the amino group at carbon 4 in the form of ammonia (NH_3), the site left by this amino group will be occupied by a water molecule. As a result, 5-methylcytosine will be completely transformed into the base thymine plus ammonia.

With high acidity, the ammonia will be converted into the ammonium ion, which can be transported as a salt to the liver, where it will be converted into urea to be excreted in the urine; and this is how the increased volume of urine in diabetics originates.

Similarly, this can happen with the intermediate compound in Figure 12, when the uracil base is being converted to its enolic form. Because upon conversion to the enolic form, carbon 5 of the uracil base becomes positive, i.e. uracil will be a Lewis acid. Therefore, when uracil is converted to the enolic form, it becomes more prone to attack by free radicals, such as the methyl group, which is introduced at carbon 5 of the enolic uracil. So, as with the cytosine base, the methyl group will be incorporated on this carbon of the enolic uracil base, and so the enolic uracil base is converted to the thymine base by methylation.

In this case, just as ammonia remains as a residue from the methylation of the cytosine base, in the methylation of the enolic uracil base, a hydrogen atom ($\frac{1}{2}H_2$) must remain free, which is then converted into a hydrogen molecule H_2. As shown in Figure 12. This is possible, as we know that molecular hydrogen is a reducing agent, which is compatible with the reducing character of homocysteine within cells.

Perhaps most importantly, the end result of the high acidity within the nucleus is that the guanine and uracil bases became enolic, and this caused the cytosine base to become thymine, as can be seen in Figure 11.

Carnivorous animals, such as hyenas, lions, dogs, tigers, cats, etc., excrete excess amino acids as allantoin via urine instead of urea. To convert these wastes to allantoin from uric acid, the enzyme urate oxidase is required. However, vegetarian animals, such as humans, do not have the enzyme urate oxidase in their excretory system; therefore, vegetarians should not eat the meat of another animal.

Fish and other marine animals excrete their cellular waste in the form of ammonia. This is because marine animals generally excrete their waste hypotonically without the need for the urinary system. Whereas birds and reptiles do not have a urinary system, because birds have to fly; and reptiles crawl on the ground. So, birds and reptiles convert their waste into uric acid and excrete it in their faeces. So, eating poultry meat does more harm because poultry meat contains more uric acid.

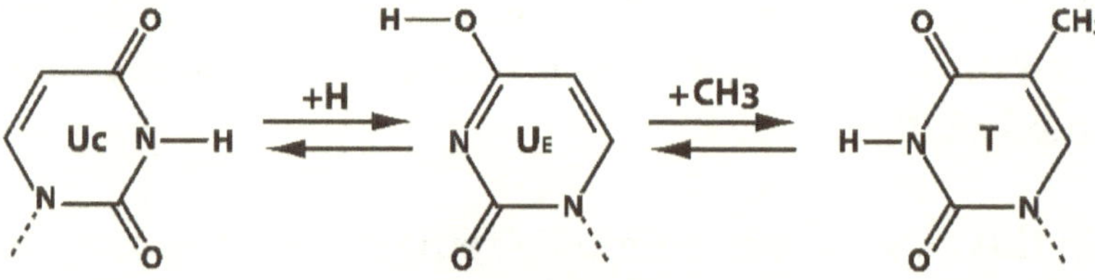

FIGURE 12

BY ACIDOSIS, THE ENOYL URACIL UE IS TRANSFORMED INTO THE THYMINE BASE T BY THE EFFECT OF METHYLATION

So, this process of methylation can happen by this way of demethylation of the amino acid methionine, which was incorporated into the cells in excess during the years of repeated consumption of animal proteins.

So, with the base pair adenine=thymine there will be no problem, because what there will be is a greater amount of thymine. With this abundance of the thymine base, the conditions for the formation of this adenine=thymine pair will be favoured, because both bases are more resistant to the increase in the degree of acidity in the cell nucleus. This adenine=thymine base pair will continue to be a natural and normal base coupling in the cell nucleus, and specifically in the chromosomes, where DNA is replicated.

The problem will arise because as the methylation process proceeds, the nucleus of that cell involved in DNA replication will at some point run out of cytosine and uracil bases. This would force the cell to chemically change the shapes of the couplings between the bases in the DNA by the chromosomes.

When the uracil base becomes enolic, this base cannot replace the cytosine base in the DNA, because the uracil base cannot form hydrogen bonds. Because there is no longer a hydrogen on the nitrogen number 3 of the enolic uracil. The only base left in the nucleus to pair with enolic guanine is thymine. Because the base thymine has a hydrogen on nitrogen 3. But there is no other base in the nucleus of the cell with these same electronic characteristics. The only base with these properties and characteristics is the thymine base.

The chemical conditions have arisen that will cause a readjustment of the electronic couplings in the DNA, which will influence the function and the original structure of that DNA; in other words, the cell mutates; and the nucleus of that cell, which is now different, will be different, because the chromosomes would use the thymine base as the other base for coupling with the guanine base, which is in enolic form. It is a coupling that normally would have been occupied by the cytosine base with the guanine base in its ketonic form but not in its enolic form; which makes it evident that the thymine base now participates with its abundance so that the chromosomes form a new type of DNA; but this DNA that the chromosomes produce will be altered with respect to the normal DNA.

As said, it will be the same in RNAs, since the uracil base is gone, and this missing uracil base will be replaced by the thymine base, which doesn't really participate normally in forming RNA. So, with this excess of the thymine base, the transfer RNA and messenger RNA can be altered, and this can influence other problems related to the sequencing of amino acids in the insertion of these in the protein chains. As we explained, the change in a nucleotide induces a change in the position of an amino acid in the protein chain; and this will contribute to the exchange of one amino acid for another; but the protein chain formed will not be the same as the one that should have been formed.

Chapter 5

SYNTHESIS ERRORS

When there is no tautomerism and methylation in the cells, the triplet that tells the ribosome where to start the synthesis of the protein chain, i.e. the initiation triplet will be as follows: uracil-adenine-cytosine (U-A-C) in the transfer RNA that must couple with the adenine-uracil-guanine ketone (A-U-Gc) triplet of the messenger RNA. Whereas, the termination triplet will be: uracil-adenine-adenine (U-A-A) in the messenger RNA, which has no amino acid in the transfer RNA; therefore, when this triplet arrives from the messenger RNA, it indicates to the ribosome that nothing goes there; that is, this triplet is what indicates to the ribosome that the synthesis of the protein chain is terminated.

When there is no cytosine or uracil in the nucleus of the cell because they have been converted to the thymine base, these triplets brought in by the messenger RNA will be different. Therefore, the insertion and amino acid sequence in the protein will be wrong. For example, the initiation triplet will be changed to: thymine-adenine-thymine (T-A-T), while the termination triplet will be thymine-adenine-adenine-adenine (T-A-A). And in this mistaken way, the ribosome will not find the code that tells it where protein synthesis will begin and how it will end.

From that moment on, both in the nucleus and in the cytoplasm of the cell, an imbalance is generated that affects the entire cell structure. The cell becomes distorted and a new kind of cell with cancerous characteristics will replicate.

Healthy, unaffected neighbouring cells will seek electronic readjustment of the chemical structure of their electronic design and functionality; and these are the cells that we must guard against an increase in acidity so that they are not outnumbered by the mutant cells. If we act in time, healthy cells will form, while cancer cells will disappear.

This will not be achieved until the healthy cell finds again its predetermined condition of acid-base concentration, which gave it an unequivocal coupling as healthy cells. In such a case, it will depend on the human being involved in the process of tautomerism and methylation, but it will not be the fault of our cells. Since we decide for ourselves what we eat and what we do not eat in order to feed our cells, which are only made of electronic matter, the cells are not aware of their existence, i.e. the mutated cells are not aware of this genetic error and only adjust to the changes imposed by the electronic charges of a chemical nature.

This is a clear example of why the magnetic mass of the spirit and the electronic matter of the body are integrated through the physical medium, but do not merge as a single genetic identity. Thus, because they are not integrated, the two entities can separate. Let us say, when the changes that happen to the electronic matter of the body culminate. This culmination is the ageing of the changes that are physical in nature. At that time of disconnection, the magnetic mass of the spirit will return to its spiritual world, while the electronic matter of the body will continue the process of change without the need for the magnetic mass of the spirit.

This electronic pairing change causes the physical and electronic configuration of the DNA to change; which will change the physical form of the electronic matter, i.e. the DNA, while this will not affect the magnetic energy of the spirit. The mass of the spirit is also unaware of the process of tautomerism and methylation.

From a physical point of view, the genome is characterised by heterogeneity and an arrangement of base pairs in the DNA. However, this arrangement of base pairs in the DNA is not random, but depends on the electronic characteristics that are formed. This is what gives the physical pattern to each individual DNA. Therefore, it is to be expected that, from this arrangement or sequence between the base pairs, a number of combinatorics will result that is really infinite in the systems of physical life.

It is the base pairs that give this combinatorial possibility, although individually the form of these pairs in DNA has to be of the form guanine-keto≡cytosine, adenine=thymine and thymine-cytokine. But, if the characteristics of these individual bonds are changed, this will influence the sequence of these base pairs in the final structure of each DNA.

For example, there are abundant regions with ketone-guanine≡cytosine triple assemblies, which is possibly the result of the more stable hydrogen bond that forms between the additional thymine-cytosine base pair, such as hydrogen bond number 3 on the left in Figure 10.

The stable three-dimensional structure of DNA will flatten out, when the enolic guanine-thymine pair is formed, because no hydrogen bond can form between the thymine-thymine pair on the right of Figure 10.

What makes DNA stable is that the ketone guanine pairs with cytosine, so that other bonds can form between the base pairs, such as the thymine-cytosine bond. The most logical way for this to happen is for the ketonic guanine-cytosine triple bond and the thymine-cytosine single pair to form between the two base pairs, which gives the DNA molecule greater energetic stability. These triple pairs are the ones that contribute the most energetic force to stabilise normal DNA. This is why the observed average content of the ketonic guanine-cytosine triple bonds is approximately 60 % higher than the theoretically expected 50 %.

Such a higher diversity of triple bonds in the order of 60 % is correlated with the so-called gene richness, which means that genes have the propensity to concentrate in those regions richer in the couplings with the ketonic guanine-keto$\equiv$cytosine triple bonds. In which case, as we can see in Figure 10, this richness of triple bonds can be diminished by the effect of acid-base alterations within the nucleus of the cells. As in the specific case of tautomerism, which influences the generation of cytokine methylation and enolic uracil.

On the left of Figure 10, you can see why in normal DNA there are preferential or more abundant regions in the triple hydrogen-bridge pairs guanine-ketonic-cytosine and thymine-cytosine. For, in such helix-shaped molecules of DNA and RNA, what exists is an interaction between electron clouds coupled according to electronic charges. Therefore, this DNA is changeable so that a rearrangement occurs; and the chemical stability of its three-dimensional structure will depend on the force of attraction with which each molecule, or groups of molecules contribute to this readjustment of the electronic charge.

The triple bonds are the ones that make the chain-like molecule twist into a spiral shape when each pair joins the ribonucleotide chain. So, the DNA chain twists to the right; which happens, as mentioned, because the sugars involved in the configuration of DNA are all of right-handed spatial configuration. So, in the left-hand strand of Figure 10, the most likely thing that can happen is that the double hydrogen bond pair appears in the adenine=thymine pair, but reversed, which will go on to make up the coding structure of that gene.

This sequence has to be completed, i.e. for the different genes to be formed, because the length of the DNA chain cannot be infinite. So, these binding forces are weakened, which means that additional pairs will not be allowed to be incorporated into the DNA sequence. This is what determines the final physical pattern of each individual DNA.

On the right hand side of Figure 10, we find the same situation, but in the wrong way due to the presence of the thymine base in the guanine-thymine enol base pair, because there is no longer any cytosine in the nucleus of the mutated cell. In this case, as we can see in Figure 10, the formation of that second hydrogen bridge between the two base pairs no longer exists. The two ketone groups of the thymine base repel each other on the wrong side of the DNA strand, causing the DNA to break open at that point. Of course, the binding strength becomes weaker in this case, so in the enol form, the binding forces will be weaker. The result is that the binding strength of the ketonic guanine-keto$\equiv$cytosine triple bond is greater than that of the enolic guanine-thymine triple bond.

So, even though a triple bond has formed between the enolic guanine/cytosine bases, this will be a less energetically stable DNA, because the thymine-cytosine bridge has not formed between the two base pairs.

Thus, its configuration will contribute less energetically to the formation of abundant zones for that gene containing the wrong pair of enolic guanine$\equiv$thymine; because this errant DNA will be energetically easier to synthesise. Although it would bring less stability with its binding strength to the DNA molecule than the normal base-pairing ketonic guanine $\equiv$cytosine did with greater strength.

DNA is what gives each organism its physical blueprint; it is the original blueprint that is established in the nucleus of each cell; it is a code; therefore, changing the structure of DNA will change the original physical blueprint with which any living thing was born. And it will always be logical, because in chemistry, the final product that results will always be the most stable, even if it is the most difficult to synthesise energetically, because what counts is the electronic stability or the lowest energy contained in the final product.

The lower energy required to form a weaker binding force will help this mutant DNA replicate faster; but, in the end, it will be a more unstable DNA compared to normal DNA. Because the linkage between the ketonic guanine$\equiv$cytosine bases incorporates greater stability into the normal DNA, compared to the case that forms with the coupling error between the enolic guanine$\equiv$thymine bases.

Once these conditions for the chromosomes to synthesise the wrong DNA have been met, the gene can lose both its sequence and its rate of replication, since the life span of each living being will depend on the speed of replication. In which case, a carrier cell with such an error will be different because of the mutant factor. Thus, a sister cell that comes from this one will also carry the same error in the future, until a large group of mutant cells is formed. As a consequence, some cells will be replicating faster than others, resulting in the formation of a lump or outgrowth of mutant cells that will become visible in the form of a tumour.

In addition, there are other kinds of genetic diseases that influence the occurrence of these inconsistencies in the archetype inherited by the human individual who has been affected by this genetic error.

The lower energetic force needed to form the enolic guanine-thymine triple bond will lighten the synthesis of that erroneous DNA, as we said; so that the presence of uracil in RNA, but not in DNA, may be a controlling chemical mechanism available to cells to accelerate the speed of protein manufacture, but at the same time to slow down the speed with which each DNA is replicated. In other words, it is this order that determines the rate at which DNA replicates in the chromosomes of the nucleus of cells in every living thing. It is what sets the pace of life.

Perhaps this is why the less energy invested in the formation of the mutated DNA will cause the mutant cells to chemically accelerate the speed of their replication, as can be seen in the accelerated growth of cancer.

This time lag makes sense from a chemical or energetic point of view, where the influencing factor is the changing character of electronic matter. Whereas, the magnetic mass of the spirit will not be altered in any way, shape or form, because the spirit is a stable form of magnetic mass; and it is independent of the electronic matter of the physical body.

These modifications imposed on the DNA of the physical body will be tolerable, as long as the number of mutant cells does not outnumber the number of healthy cells. So, that the whole organism does not collapse permanently. As it turns out, the cellular body will not be able to withstand this accelerated growth of mutant cells for long, because this functionality, which is logical from a chemical point of view, does not correspond to the same conditions as the human being that was originally formed.

The distorted process can be reversed, but only if the person realises that the cancer problem is of a chemical nature, and if he can change his or her dietary strategy in time. In this case, the magnetic mass of the spirit will not be disconnected from the electronic matter of the body, but the spirit will be enhanced by this knowledge, which is the only thing it will be able to take back with it when it is time to return to its spiritual world. That is to say, only the knowledge of its chemical process will enhance the magnetic mass of the spirit.

The spirit cannot take anything containing electronic matter back to its spirit world; for the spirit consists only of magnetic mass without any electronic matter whatsoever. So, there is no point in accumulating material fortunes on earth but a wealth of knowledge.

Such modifications may not be tolerated by the original genome of the germ cells, so that the modifications acquired by the individual who modified them will be passed on to his offspring. This goes some way to explaining why some of these readjustments or mutations occur continuously, and why the appearance of the beings is changing for the better. But these modifications must be greater in human beings, because what we observe is that there are many forms of human beings within the same race.

That is why, at present, the number of diseases due to these continuous genetic modifications is in the order of 4,000.

The most common being cystic fibrosis. However, very little is known about this relationship with the hereditary nature of cancer, but only moderate changes that manifest themselves in those generations that inherit them.

But cancer is not hereditary. The non-hereditary nature of cancer is demonstrated by Dr. Paul Liechtenstein of the Department of Medical Epidemiology at the Karolinska Institute. A university medical institution in Sweden.

Dr. Liechtenstein analysed the clinical cases of 44,788 homozygous twins, i.e. individuals who share an identical genetic configuration. For the data analysis, cases from medical records of twins who died of cancer from Swedish, Danish and Finnish death registries were studied in order to assess the statistics of having malignant tumours in 28 different parts of the body. In each of the registers, the medical records of twins born between 1886 and 1958 were analysed. Between 1926 and 1958 alone, more than half of just one of the twins had died from some form of cancer.

The analysis should have concluded that the other twin of the brother or sister affected by cancer of the stomach, colon, lung, breast or prostate, etc., had the same risk of suffering from the same disease due to genetic similarity. However, the result was that the genetic factors provided little evidence of the likelihood of both twins being prone to developing the same type of cancer.

It is the chemical environment within the cells that plays a critical role in the likelihood of one twin having this abnormality, because whether or not the twins get cancer depends on their dietary lifestyle. For it is the way we eat that leads us to alter the acid-base balance inside and outside the cells.

Continuing with methylation. In December 2007, one of the members of the British Whitehead Laboratory research group, Rudolf Jaenisch, demonstrated that there is a link between the phenomenon of methylation and the development of colon tumours in mice. For them, methylation is the accumulation of excess methyl groups in certain parts of DNA. They were able to deduce that methylation causes the deactivation of the gene that monitors the correct functioning of DNA, or that this is the gene that has the job of repairing or reversing what could be the start of a genetic error, and as a consequence, incites the formation of small polyps. Methylation was also found to increase the frequency of intestinal tumours in mice by 60-100%, and on average significantly increases the growth of microscopic tumours.

DNA methylation has been correlated with the development of cancerous tumours in humans, as it is a type of chemical modification in DNA that can be inherited, provided the modification is tolerable.

This would explain why cancer occurs in children who have not eaten enough meat at a young age. But in this case, the methylation was inherited from the mother. Because it is a mutation inherited from the gestation of the diploid, it will be more difficult to reverse it chemically, as it is part of the whole genetic conglomerate of the child. These altered genes function by chemical logic, but are biologically dislocated.

Whereas normally, in a person born healthy, the genetic error could be repaired without appreciable changes in the original DNA sequence. But only the intervention of the cell's own natural chemical environment is necessary. One can help to achieve this relief by returning to a vegetarian lifestyle, i.e., by consuming plant foods that are suitable for the cellular framework of a human being.

The opportunity could be given for the cellular system to return to its normal acidity or pH conditions. In other words, this process of reversing methylation and tautomerism would be what causes the progression of cancer to be chemically interrupted on its own, since the cells have the mechanisms and their own action to correct themselves for these anomalies, which we have induced through our own fault.

How? By regularising the consumption of sugar in the form of sucrose, dairy products, vegetables rich in oxalic acid and fizzy drinks, as the enzyme carbonic anhydrase will convert the carbon dioxide contained in fizzy drinks into carbonic acid. Definitely refrain from eating meat of any kind until the accelerated growth of the mutated cells can be stopped. If you want to remain a carnivore, the same cancer-related afflictions are bound to recur.

So, this effect of healthy eating is what regulates a normal process to occur through the mechanism of genetic modification, because it also requires adaptive activity of certain genes in those inherited regions of the genome, depending on what the cells need to express or do at any given time.

As all cells that make up the same organism possess a configuration of bases in the DNA that are identical, the covert sequence of that DNA will be a key element for the identity to be inherited by the future cell.

This process, or having different kinds of cells with different activities, is what is known as cell differentiation, since all these cells originated from a diploid. This would be a logical and necessary multitude of mutations from stem cells, as long as the bases in the DNA are not swapped, as only the sequence of genes must be altered to produce other forms of life, or a wide variety of distinctive cells found in the body of a human being.

Also, mutation is a natural and necessary reason for the improvement and perfection of each race. For example, every day more beautiful women and more intelligent children are born. The qualities for the behaviour of each being come in their magnetic memory. But, from the physical point of view, these will be the most capable men and women to contribute to the physical improvement of their race.

Physical behaviour is different from psychological behaviour. Psychological behaviour is an activity which has its origin in the magnetic mass. This psychological behaviour is an instinct of insects such as ants and bees, or animals who compete with each other, and only the female and male who have a higher energetic force, and therefore a higher genetic and psychological capacity for the betterment of their race, will remain.

This means that when a cell divides, this cell will be able to transmit to its descendant cell that improvement or actualisation of its physical pattern. But the original behaviour of the spirit is embodied in the magnetic mass. Therefore, this quality cannot disappear by the disconnection of the spirit from the physical body, for the two kinds of energy cannot be separated. They do not disappear in the same way that tautomerism and methylation disappear, because tautomerism and methylation are qualities that belong to the electronic matter of the physical body.

The natural methylation, characteristics and sequential pattern must be maintained in the harmony and genetic memory of the physical matter of the living being, because the magnetic mass of the spirit is the energy that gives life form to the physical electronic matter. Therefore, in the physical world, the information must be maintained in the new cell that is to be formed. For example, if the new cell that originates belongs to the heart, the cells that are formed must maintain the function of their progenitors in order to inherit the same instructions on how to contract and dilate in order to continue the work of ejecting blood.

But if the cell is modified by tautomerism and methylation, the functioning characteristics of the electronic matter of the physical body will be lost, and the new cell that emerges will no longer be able to perform the same function as its ancestor. The correct sequence of guanine-keto, cytosine, thymine and adenine bases in the cell's DNA is what allows these bases to replicate without error, but they must also carry the instructions that must appear in the new cell that is formed.

In cells, as mentioned, it is the ribosomes that carry out the task of protein synthesis, and similar to the example of reading a text with spelling mistakes, the ribosome has to recognise and analyse that sequence properly, to try to minimise the probability of introducing an error, which could lead to the wrong result of confusion and function with respect to the appropriate proteins produced by healthy cells. This process of ribosome and cell nucleus function depends on the degree of acidity within the cell, but more specifically within the cell nucleus. It is worth mentioning that the Golgi apparatus is the organelle that inspects the functionality of the proteins produced in the ribosomes.

Let's say, this was a very careful analysis, to know how our cells function, and what is the kind of energy that makes them function to give mobility to all living beings; that is, so that electronic matter can be transformed into other forms of electronic matter, and can be used by the magnetic mass of the spirit in order to give the form of life to every being, in this physical station of the Earth.

Our only intention with this series of books is to explain how the Universe began; and that the Universe is the creator of the energy and all that exists in the Universe, with the purpose that humanity changes its way of thinking and acting; since, due to the lack of knowledge of its origin, the human being is destroying himself, the forest and all the animals, which perhaps have no notion of their existence, but have feelings. Because it is urgent to act in time to save the animals and the planet Earth from the disintegration of life.

REGARDING THE AUTHOR'S WORK

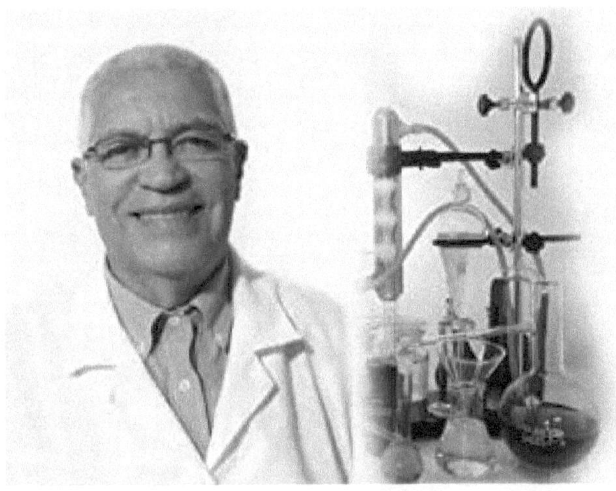

Graduated from the School of Chemistry, Faculty of Sciences, Universidad Central de Venezuela, with a degree in Chemical Technology. Postgraduate studies in Food Science and Technology. Special work on the chemistry of natural products and the chemistry of diseases. Chemical process designer. Books you can locate on Amazon.com®. These books must be subject to revision as we clarify how the Universe was formed: "The Chemistry of Cancer". "The Chemistry of Diabetes. "The Heart Attack". "Alzheimer's". "The Chemistry of Arthritis". "The Chemistry of Thought". "The Chemistry of the Spirit". "How the Universe was formed". "The Expensalists". "Why You Shouldn't Eat Meat". "The Micro World". "Does God Really Exist?". "Objecting to Albert Einstein's Relativity". "Divining the Future". "The Mistake of the Great Scientists". "Life on the Sun". "The Universe before Zero Time". "The Energy of the Spirit". "The Origin of Cancer". "The World of Cells". "The Chemistry of Disease". "The Particle that Created the Universe". The Chemistry of Cancer, seventh edition. The Chemistry of Diabetes sixth edition; The Chemistry of Heart Attack fourth edition, "The Chemistry of Memory"; The Chemistry of Arthritis third edition. "The Creative Power of the Mind. The Particle that Formed the Universe, third edition. "The Initial Mass of the Universe". "You Shouldn't Eat Meat". "The Origin of the Body and the Spirit". "Worship the Universe". "Sugar an

Enemy in the Kitchen". "Time Travel". The Chemistry of Diabetes, Issue 7. The Chemistry of Heart Attack Issue 5. The Memory of the Spirit Issue 1, The Chemistry of Arthritis Issue 5. "The Starting Point of the Universe" The Particle that Created the Universe Issue 5 "The Evolution of Spirit". "The Life of Spirit". "Rewriting Science". "The Beginning of the Universe". "Spiritual Growth". "Coupling of the Spirit with the Body". "The Origin of Life". "The Particle that Created the Universe, Issue 8". "Death Does Not Exist".